Joshua Tambe

Medical research for beginners

Joshua Tambe

Medical research for beginners

Perspectives and a novel approach

LAP LAMBERT Academic Publishing

Impressum / Imprint

Bibliografische Information der Deutschen Nationalbibliothek: Die Deutsche Nationalbibliothek verzeichnet diese Publikation in der Deutschen Nationalbibliografie; detaillierte bibliografische Daten sind im Internet über http://dnb.d-nb.de abrufbar.

Alle in diesem Buch genannten Marken und Produktnamen unterliegen warenzeichen-, marken- oder patentrechtlichem Schutz bzw. sind Warenzeichen oder eingetragene Warenzeichen der jeweiligen Inhaber. Die Wiedergabe von Marken, Produktnamen, Gebrauchsnamen, Handelsnamen, Warenbezeichnungen u.s.w. in diesem Werk berechtigt auch ohne besondere Kennzeichnung nicht zu der Annahme, dass solche Namen im Sinne der Warenzeichen- und Markenschutzgesetzgebung als frei zu betrachten wären und daher von jedermann benutzt werden dürften.

Bibliographic information published by the Deutsche Nationalbibliothek: The Deutsche Nationalbibliothek lists this publication in the Deutsche Nationalbibliografie; detailed bibliographic data are available in the Internet at http://dnb.d-nb.de.

Any brand names and product names mentioned in this book are subject to trademark, brand or patent protection and are trademarks or registered trademarks of their respective holders. The use of brand names, product names, common names, trade names, product descriptions etc. even without a particular marking in this work is in no way to be construed to mean that such names may be regarded as unrestricted in respect of trademark and brand protection legislation and could thus be used by anyone.

Coverbild / Cover image: www.ingimage.com

Verlag / Publisher:
LAP LAMBERT Academic Publishing
ist ein Imprint der / is a trademark of
OmniScriptum GmbH & Co. KG
Heinrich-Böcking-Str. 6-8, 66121 Saarbrücken, Deutschland / Germany
Email: info@lap-publishing.com

Herstellung: siehe letzte Seite /
Printed at: see last page
ISBN: 978-3-659-25830-5

Copyright © 2015 OmniScriptum GmbH & Co. KG
Alle Rechte vorbehalten. / All rights reserved. Saarbrücken 2015

Contents

Dedication ...... *iii*

Foreword ...... *iv*

Preface ...... *v*

Acknowledgements ...... *vi*

Chapter One. Medical trainees and research: Perspectives 7

    Visibility of end-of-course medical research projects 9

    Interest in research by medical trainees 11

Chapter Two. Case study: Experience of a cohort of medical trainees 15

    Perspectives 15

    Appraisal of a novel self-help tool 17

Chapter Three. The "art" and the "science" of medicine 20

Chapter Four. Research: What medical trainees ought to know 22

    Research as a career 24

    Experiences of some beginners in research 26

    Two vital questions 27

    Getting started 27

Chapter Five. A novel self-help tool 30

    Model template 31

    Seven Steps 34

Chapter Six. Organizing ideas 53

Title of the project 53

　　　Abstract 54

　　　Description of the project 54

Chapter Seven. Appraising evidence 61

　　　Research question(s), hypotheses; are they clear? 61

　　　Study design; appropriate? 61

　　　Methods; well described? 64

　　　Data presentation; correct summary statistics? 64

　　　What measures of disease frequency and association? 67

　　　Role of chance, bias, and confounding addressed? 68

　　　Statistical tests 69

　　　Data interpretation 69

　　　Study conclusion(s) based on findings or intuitive? 75

　　　Your own conclusion 75

Bibliography 77

To Arabella,

Clarence, Caleb and Caren

Foreword

Individuals who choose to pursue the medical profession live with the privilege and responsibility of providing life changing counsel to patients. However, the medical profession is always changing. Every year, there are new diagnostic strategies, new treatments, new preventive strategies and new ways of delivering information. It is therefore imperative for medical professionals to stay abreast with current evidence, or better still generate their own locally relevant evidence by conducting research, with the ultimate aim of providing high quality care to their patients.

Medical research is not often the focus of medical training and many trainees or professionals are overwhelmed with the daunting task of posing an answerable research question, designing a study, conducting said study with high standards and reporting accordingly.

The next chapters offer resources to guide less experienced medical researchers through the process. Potential researchers are invited to reflect upon the purpose and goals of their research and how to go about it. Additional resources are discussed for those who crave for more knowledge, and in the event that all else fails the most invaluable piece of advice still stands – consult an expert.

Happy reading!

Lawrence Mbuagbaw, MD, MPH, PhD, FRSPH

Hamilton, Canada, 2015

Preface

Many medical students get engaged in research activities during their final year of medical studies. Others only get to do so during postgraduate training whilst some – yes, they never! It is important for health care providers to understand basic research principles to be able to critically appraise scientific evidence and follow guidelines during clinical practice. Getting into research for the first time as a final-year medical student is a great and sometimes frustrating experience for many especially in settings without a strong research culture. There are many final-year trainees who have research topics but do not really understand what they are "doing". Plagiarism of dissertations, theses and/or journal articles with a similar focus is common practice. This is of course an easier and feasible option as it might go unnoticed.

As a beginner in research it is possible to pick up a research topic and "make sense" out of it without much external help. That is the purpose for this book. Writing a research proposal/protocol can be a daunting task for anyone making his/her debut in research. A self-help tool tailored to meet the needs of trainees in the clinical sciences is presented to help guide the beginner through this process. Its development was inspired by the desire of a former medical trainee to assist those in need (*Hebrews 2:18*). Other research concepts are briefly explained when encountered in an effort to provide a one-stop-shop source of information where necessary. It is hoped it serves the need for which it is intended.

Joshua Tambe

Brussels, April 2015

Acknowledgements

I am grateful to the many teachers, mentors, colleagues, students, and friends who in some way have influenced my training and career pursuits.

My family has been an immense source of inspiration.

THANK YOU.

Chapter One

Medical trainees and research: Perspectives

Introduction

Research activities are mandatory requirements for certification in some medical schools in different countries. In such schools final-year medical trainees at both undergraduate and postgraduate levels are expected to submit a piece of research work to be evaluated and graded by academic staff. Some schools further plan for and organize a public defense of end-of-course research projects. The impact of a research project is such that it can contribute to up to 50% of the total score in some medical schools. It is therefore a strong determinant of the final grades in the transcript of some medical trainees. Consequently it should receive sufficient attention by both students and academic staff. But how much importance it is given remains a cause for concern. Imposing dissertations or theses for certification is one thing, creating and sustaining a strong research culture is another.

Engaging in research is a brand-new experience from routine lectures in classrooms and bed-side clinical rounds. Many students often embrace it with mixed feelings. This is so because they often do not know what to expect from this "new course". Some of us got involved in research activities for the first time in our final-year in medical school. And so it is for many medical students who get excited during didactic lectures on research methodology and impatiently wait to get started on a research project that will give them the opportunity to apply what they have learned. They then dream of a brilliant and stunning presentation in front of academic staff, course-mates, friends and family members on the day of the public defense. This is however not the case for some other students who remain entirely skeptical about the usefulness of such an exercise.

It is expected that these end-of-course research projects for medical trainees would serve as a foundation for the acquisition of basic skills in research. These skills would probably be used sometime later in their career as they seek to provide health care for those who chose to restrict themselves to clinical practice. For others who intend to get into research as a career these skills would serve as a framework to build on. But these are expectations from academic policies. The fruitfulness of this policy of mandatory research activities for medical trainees can be ascertained through divers means. One of these can be through the quality of research work produced and the impact these works have. Another means can be through the production of career researchers as a result of initiation and mentoring into research.

Regarding research quality, this can be assessed through publications in peer-reviewed scientific journals which publish academic works of commendable quality and standards. The impact of a research project in informing decisions and policies also attests of its relevance and quality (though not always). If there is a strong research culture in a society then it is likely this will also produce many more "converts" who will definitely mature into full-blown researchers.

It is possible for medical trainees to carry out research and publish in scientific journals of high standing even as students. They do not need to be career researchers for this, and this kind of engagement is encouraged by some academic institutions. In fact some researchers have reported an increase in research articles published by medical students over a period of time, while noting that these articles were hardly ever made reference to in other academic works.[1] Some also noted continuous encouragement of medical trainees' research activities was associated with a positive outcome, including more self-confidence and motivation to pursue a career in research.[2,3] However this type of encouragement is lacking in many other settings.

There is however sufficient reason to believe that end-of-course research activities are gradually becoming mere routine or just some form of academic formality for many. Research skills development and career orientation have been given less importance. The research exercise is the last "hurdle" to leave school and get into practice. This situation is regrettable and unfortunate as it undermines the usefulness of the very process that generates the knowledge that should guide current practice and which will inform future practice.

Visibility of end-of-course medical research projects

An increase in enrolment in medical schools will result to a corresponding increase in the number of end-of-course research projects. If all of these projects were to result in scientific publications this would boost the publication output of many medical faculties.

Some researchers have taken interest in investigating the information products of end-of-course research projects in different medical schools around the world at both undergraduate and postgraduate levels. Results from some studies carried out in Europe, South America, the Middle East, Asia and Africa provide overwhelming evidence that a significant number of end-of-course medical research projects do not result in publications in indexed scientific journals.[4-7]

These research projects are therefore likely to have been published in journals that do not have much visibility or are covered with dust in some university library. One may ask: Why aren't the findings of these studies disseminated to a wider scientific community? Why would students and their supervisors choose to "bury" the findings of their research project in one school library where it would be accessible only to a very limited number of persons? This might raise concerns on the relevance and quality of such projects. Was there really a sound rationale for some of these research projects? Were the methods appropriate? Did the studies actually measure what they purported? Were the projects commensurate with the level of the certificate for which they were being carried out? Were the studies actually carried out? These are just some of the many questions one may ask to understand why results of studies would not be disseminated.

However to make available the research findings of academic projects, some universities now deposit theses and dissertations in some online databases. This is a commendable initiative.

It might be said that the type of journal can be used as a proxy to assess the quality of a published paper. Perhaps not always. Nevertheless high-quality peer-review has an undeniable role in improving upon the quality of any academic work. But papers only get to peer-reviewers after they must have survived editorial screening! Editorial policies may be such that most submitted manuscripts get turned away almost immediately. Rigorous peer-reviews are also often merciless to papers deemed unsatisfactory, uninteresting and below standard. After a couple of rejections the paper then finds a suitable home, probably local this time and often without the stress of going through a rigorous peer-review process. There is a home for every paper, some say. Consequently electronic searches for articles in journal-indexing databases using filters such as "peer-review" will not identify such studies. If those papers are retrieved manually they might not be included for synthesis and analysis in review articles as they would be judged to be of "insufficient" quality as a result of the filter.

Some researchers have reported a high rate of plagiarism in some end-of-course medical research projects.[8] Large sections of other documents such as journal articles and previous theses and dissertations were reproduced in some of these projects. This is a cause for concern and supposes some grave defects in the knowledge of scientific writing by these new "authors". Probably these trainees were abandoned to themselves to work without proper supervision and final copies of project reports (theses, dissertations) were never sufficiently proof-read. Local supervisors have a big role to play on the quality of the projects they supervise. Institutional policies if strong enough can further reinforce quality and abort some projects before they ever get to term to tarnish the image or reputation of these institutions. Such findings are disheartening and further put into question the credibility of some research projects and entire academic systems. No wonder much of these products never find their way into scientific platforms which promote sound research and advocate for quality.

Interest in research by medical trainees

Many studies have reported a lack of interest in research by medical students and residents in very different settings.[9,10] The motivation is low and there is very little or no will to engage into research activities (but obliged to do so in schools where a research project is mandatory). Whatever the basis for their views it is curious to find out that some even consider end-of-course research projects to be of very little value to their training, not to say completely worthless. This indifference to research by trainees in a scientific knowledge-driven discipline is quite regrettable and demonstrates how much academic systems have failed to inculcate into future practitioners the value of the process that shapes what they know and will be practicing.

Several reasons, some of which are advanced by trainees could explain this delusion.[11] Some say lectures have not been helpful or comprehensive. These lectures have been too theoretical and abstract without much link to what the trainees hope to be doing as main activity after graduating from school. The value of research in future practice is not emphasized and so it is therefore considered as one of those "optional" modules, implying the knowledge and skills are not a necessity. Observations show that often courses on research methods can be very infrequent in some school curricula and only thought of when a cohort of students gets to their final year of studies.

Supervision, guidance and mentoring have also been described as inadequate or quasi-inexistent by some medical trainees. Some trainees say their research experience was or actually is a bad one and they would either not want to remember or are just praying and hoping it all comes to an end soonest. It appears research project supervisors always seem to expect much from where nothing or very little has been sown.

Facilities for research often appear to be completely absent, inadequate or obsolete. Inappropriate, archaic or absent equipments, the lack of academic resources, no or low levels of funding, the lack of motivation, a drain of skilled and competent staff with an overall poor organizational culture have taken hostage entire academic systems. How then can quality be expected? Through what means? Would the level of the trainees not serve as a proxy of the level and performance of the trainers in a given system? It sure does.

Many other factors can be identified, some of which are specific to particular contexts. However these factors often coexist and it can be difficult to separate the effect of any one of them from the others. It is therefore necessary to adopt a holistic approach, study the interactions of individual predictors and plan for interventions to improve upon this situation if long-lasting solutions are ever envisaged.

If we consider that often research topics are handed to medical trainees by prospective supervisors without their input to be later coached on it, we may understand why commitment might not be optimal. Generally people are more committed doing what they love and enjoy. This is not any different when it comes to research. They do not get bored easily, can dedicate several hours working on it and will do everything to look for solutions when problems arise. This is intrinsic motivation, and might not be the case when literally "dragged" into a research topic because trainees have not been prepared for anything over the years or previous attempts at other ambitious projects have not yielded positive results and the academic timetable is catching up with them.

During such stressful situations what can be expected of them? Often they are unfamiliar with scientific writing and have never participated in research activities. They now have to run behind potential supervisors who offer them hope, follow directives whether they understand or not, do some reading on some topic they are likely to be unfamiliar with and less inspired about, assemble related material from anywhere and build up a dissertation or thesis. One motivation now drives the student, and that is to also have "something" to present as an end-of-course research project and be gone.

In my opinion if mentored into a discipline and carefully guided during training, potential fields for research can become obvious even before a research project as partial fulfillment for certification might be required by the institution if that is the case. In this way trainees can get attracted to some disciplines and start developing interest in carrying out research which will help them further understand some concepts. It is very likely this kind of early mentorship into research activities will be more fruitful and initiate the trainee into the world of scientific and academic writing. Further encouragement might just be what would be needed to get the trainee make giant strides into academic writing, seek to continuously improve and sharpen their skills and definitely cruise over final-year research projects. We could then be sure a researcher would be in the making. These are the trainees more likely to get into academic careers and excel. The love for research would have been born, nurtured and allowed to develop through active participation in different many research projects. Research activities would not be burdensome or become a "necessary evil" because of academic advancement. The importance of research would be appreciated and embraced, and this devotion and love for it might just be what would be needed to produce quality and mentor other trainees into research, taking into account of course a favorable environment.

Chapter Two

Case study: Experience of a cohort of medical trainees

Perspectives

A few years of assistance to medical students and residents at different stages of their end-of-course research projects made some difficulties very apparent. It was clear many had some real problems and the observed level of understanding of research concepts varied immensely. Some trainees (few though) were quite knowledgeable and required just guidance, others could actually be brought to understand some principles whilst some were at a complete loss about almost everything – not even the basics.

It was however thought necessary to survey the opinion of a cohort of final-year medical trainees working on their research projects to have an idea of their experiences. This survey was therefore aimed at identifying their needs and possible explanations for their experiences. The usefulness of didactic lectures from the trainees' point of view and the identification of areas that would need to be improved were specifically assessed. Notwithstanding, such a survey would also give an idea of the level of support from academic staff the trainees who participated in the survey received.

The survey was carried out in a pioneer medical school in Cameroon after ethical and administrative clearance was obtained.[12] The study population, made up of final-year undergraduate and postgraduate medical trainees working on their end-of course research projects was identified. Consenting participants filled the study questionnaire. This questionnaire was standardized and pilot-tested using a cohort comprised of a previous batch of medical trainees of the same institution. Further details on the methods can be found in a published article.[12]

The findings from this survey confirmed previous observations but also brought out other issues.[13,14] Just about one out of ten had been involved in previous research activities leading to a scientific publication. Well, not much would be expected from undergraduates at this level as just 4% reported being a coauthor in a scientific article. But 10% for postgraduates who obligatorily carried out an undergraduate thesis? That means most of the studies were not published. Peer-review was not used as a filter to assess any reported published paper, leaving concerns that the percentage might have been lower.

Every single participant reported having benefitted from lectures on research methods. Nevertheless the value of some of these lectures were downplayed by most undergraduate students (87%) according to whom these lectures were insufficient or did not contain anything to help them in their research projects and so very much still had to get real help from somewhere else. Postgraduate trainees had a better appreciation for lectures on research methods. It is likely that previous research experience at undergraduate level improved the receptiveness for postgraduate trainees.

Some difficulties were raised up again and again by the trainees at both levels, suggesting that these concepts were considerable obstacles and emphasis would be required during lectures to consolidate understanding. Based on the frequency of occurrences of each difficulty, they are presented subsequently in descending order of magnitude. Adopting and efficiently using a referencing style topped the list, followed by the lack of clues for the write-up of a research protocol. Not knowing where to look up related relevant material for the literature review and being at a loss to figure out *a priori* statistical methods that could be employed in their projects were also expressed as concerns. Finally the making of a data collection sheet, drafting of questionnaires and writing up a methodology were also cited as difficulties. If many could have such difficulties then this could be used as a proxy to assess the quality and impact of some didactic lectures on research methods. If these lectures were really insufficient as was claimed then it would not be surprising that slightly less than fifty percent of respondents did consider end-of-course research activities as really necessary.

In my opinion, early initiation into research courses and activities can be a good starting point to create interest in medical trainees.[15,16] Course contents should be assessed and improved continuously. There should be adequate hands-on research training with emphasis on concepts directly related to medical practice for trainees to easily grasp the importance of scientific methods. Supervision and mentoring should be improved and the necessary infrastructures should be put in place. Also, academic writing can be encouraged and rewarded during medical training. It might be worthwhile elucidating and implementing proper selection criteria for academic staff and they should be constantly trained and assessed in settings where this is not common practice. Many other solutions can be envisaged depending on the prevailing local socio-economic and political situation of each setting.

Appraisal of a novel self-help tool

With an understanding of the difficulties some medical trainees were experiencing with end-of-course research projects, it was thought that an "outline" or some kind of "checklist" might be necessary to help them determine by themselves if they were on course. Not only do some have topics and do not know what to do with them, there are those who have actually made a write-up but cannot give a simple or plain language summary of what they had done! This would suppose the trainee does not fully understand the purpose and methods of their research.

Once a set of points was written down and checked for coherence, this was handed to some research amateurs seeking help to assess their research projects all by themselves. The reaction was immediate. There were comments like "I think I now know what to do", "I'll have to rearrange my work and make things clear", "I missed out on many things", "This is inspirational", etc.

It was then decided to test the set of points using a wider group of trainees at both undergraduate and postgraduate levels irrespective of what their research topics were to assess the usefulness of this "checklist" in guidance and to investigate potential difficulties. Pre-testing was done using English and French versions of this set of points which was later modified and then christened a "model template". Especially some hints were added (see template in Chapter Five) after pre-testing since the objective was to produce a self-help tool that was supposed to be easy-to-use. The testing of the template constituted the second part of a survey. Participants were offered a printed copy of the template and blank sheets of papers. They were instructed to read through the template carefully, then to use the different steps for guidance and elucidate their research topics. Ideas had to be written on the blank sheets of paper provided (which they had to keep to preserve their ideas). After this exercise some questions followed on the questionnaire, permitting the participants to appraise the template.

This tool was appreciated by the study participants who accepted to work on it using their research topics. Guidance and clarity of their work stood out as the first major high-point. Some declared they now understood what they had to do with their topics after using the tool, as they could explain it in plain language. The template was easy to use independently even though help from the principal investigator was readily available if it was thought necessary. Developed to be used as a self-help tool meant the expected level of difficulty had to be low and this was reported so. Respondents were under no pressure to work in front of the investigator or assess the tool immediately to hand in their responses. The aim was to assess the usefulness of a novel tool and not the ability of the student to use it. So despite the fact that the study outcomes were not blinded, it was in the best interest of the trainees to objectively report their experience.

These trainees had been exposed to didactic lectures on research methods at some point of their training, and so this could have facilitated the use of this novel tool, reason for which I believe this tool is not to be used as a standalone but rather as an adjunct to lectures on research methods.

Chapter Three

The "art" and the "science" of medicine

Do medical trainees and practitioners need to carry out research? It is not the main line of their activities, some argue. Of what benefit will research activities and publications be to them? Of course much if they have a university career! But for those who are not in *academia*? How will it impact patient care or routine daily practice for clinicians? These are some of the questions about medical practice and research that raise some controversies on the focus of training and curricula development.

The demonstration of professional skills and competence by medical practitioners during interactions with their clients is an art. It can be taught and learned, but to a large extent depends on personal characteristics of individual practitioners. Good technical knowledge complementing these virtues will produce a good practitioner. **This is the art of medicine** (*and the basis for evidence!*)

The knowledge base for much of medical practice is generated through scientific methods.[17] This knowledge however does not impose itself on the practitioner, but the latter will always judge if the knowledge can be applied to the particular situation at hand and to what extent. This is application of scientific evidence. **Medicine is therefore an applied science** (*evidence-based!*)

The scientific methods that generate scientific knowledge to help guide medical decisions are often observed during routine practice, and it is therefore necessary that the medical practitioner should have mastery of the principles involved. S/he can therefore produce information that will serve as the basis for evidence in decision-making in their practice.

The knowledge guiding clinical practice cannot just be totally dependent on subjective observations and personal experience. In my opinion physicians have to be trained to have a strong scientific background. Otherwise:

- How can we expect quality care if the very basis for evidence is not understood?
- How reliable can clinical decisions be if not based on some form of evidence?

If medical trainees do not get acquainted with scientific methods, there will be questions as to whether they will be in a position to effectively scrutinize any form of scientific evidence. Critical appraisal skills are important in judging the quality of scientific knowledge. Medicine is very much an art and an applied science, and as Panda wrote: "To be a good medical practitioner, one has to become a good artist with sufficient scientific knowledge".[18]

Chapter Four

Research: What medical trainees ought to know

If a researcher can successfully come up with a feasible and elaborate strategy that permits correct data collection for their study, then they would have done the essential. If you are good in statistics and data analysis these would be an added advantage, otherwise expert assistance can be requested. Sophisticated analytical procedures will not improve on the quality of poor data resulting from a flawed process, as the adage goes "garbage in, garbage out".

It is not easy to appreciate the complexities involved in carrying out research just from lectures on research methods. These are best ascertained through active participation in designing and conducting many research projects. Almost every research project differs in some way from another, and the subtle aspects responsible for these differences are not easily understood or picked up by the uninitiated. It is difficult to sufficiently explain in a classroom the dynamism in knowledge application involved in designing different research projects. Didactic lectures are often rich with hypothetical examples after which it is assumed the student has understood the underlying principles. Only when actively involved in the designing and conduct of a research project can a student really appreciate the content of lectures on research methods.

Complex problems arising during research activities can be frustrating to students (especially if they are ill-prepared for research). At times talking about these difficulties to fellow students as is often the case doesn't help as these other students are probably working on something entirely different and so do not even understand what is being talked about! Worse still the project supervisor might not be readily available or accessible. Things are not made any easier for the student when initial drafts of the manuscript, a product of countless hours of reading and consultations are harshly described as "rubbish" and "fit for the bin".

It is unfortunate that some medical schools do not have a strong research culture and medical trainees are not adequately supervised either because university and hospital staffs are over-burdened, insufficient, or there is the lack of infrastructure. Consequently the research experience is burdensome and trainees hardly ever get to really understand research principles. Some make use of former dissertations or theses in libraries, reproducing subsequent sections or chapters "as is" without any consideration of relevance. Are you a final-year student who is pondering over a research project but yet do not have a clear idea of what you really want to do? Or do you have a research topic already but do not know where to begin? If you ever went through this ordeal or are actually doing so then rest assured that you are simply going through what other researchers (even some of the most successful) have gone through! Your difficulties and fears are not unique to you. Do not be worried.

That is how research often looks like when you begin. Many begin research without a very clear idea of what they really want to do. They have a "hazy" view of the "big picture". As a beginner it is quite difficult being as clear as print when you begin a research project.

If you are about to carry out a research project and you do not have a very clear idea of what you want to do, do not be worried. Just stay on.

Research methodology is taught following an orderly and coherent sequence (as expected), but you see practical application often does not *always* follow that order! Perhaps nobody ever told you that. Nobody really tells you the objectives of their remarkable study were redefined after all the data had been collected and analyzed. Nobody tells you that the final methodology was carefully written after data collection and analysis. Yet the initial samples were discarded and the first questionnaires were dumped after pre-testing. Even the title of that well-written article you consider reproducing in your own setting, published in a world-renowned peer-reviewed international journal was formulated after the entire manuscript had been drafted and proof-read a couple of times.

Yes! It is true. All you see is the final product, a colorful and neatly written paper published in a "prestigious" international scientific journal! How did the authors get there? That is the puzzle you will have to learn to solve as a beginner in research. Not a difficult one though, but one that can scare you away from the onset. This approach is employed or has been used at one point by many researchers (will they admit?) It is not the "gold standard" of scientific research and I am not advocating for it. *However, the beginner in research should be aware that most things appear clearer retrospectively.* After going through an exercise you can better appreciate the experience. With active participation in different research projects the amateur researcher gets sharpened, becomes mature and can better appreciate good science.

Research as a career

Simply put, research can be said to be the systematic collection, analysis and interpretation of information in order to generate knowledge. This knowledge will be used to inform policies and decision-making. Information gathered today will serve as the basis for what we will do tomorrow and while doing it we gather information on how what we do is performing, and use that information to further modify the way we should do it in the near future.

The world is ever-changing and so is technology, resources, the way people behave, etc. There is the need to continuously study "processes" in an ever-changing environment. What worked yesterday might not work today due to the introduction of some factors that were not present yesterday or a change in others, and what is working today might not work tomorrow for a similar reason. So it is important to constantly seek and apply knowledge for continuous improvement. Some with no idea of what research is all about dare to wonder aloud why researchers never seem to "find what they are looking for!"

You really do not need to be a career researcher to carry out research. Studying your own environment, behavior, attitudes and making adjustments is research! This basic understanding of research is important for everyone to grasp. Governments, institutions, companies, businessmen, other professionals, and even students change strategies based on prior experiences and predictable patterns. These changes in strategies and decisions are part of everyday life so basically everyone is carrying out research continuously, even without being consciously aware of that. Whatever view people hold concerning research, its value in shaping knowledge and society cannot be ignored.

Principles underlying scientific research

An important difference between the knowledge that informs your decisions in everyday life and the knowledge from scientific studies is based on the way both are generated. An event, experience, or information from any source can be used as the basis of knowledge for an individual to make any decision at any time. However in scientific research there is often a kind of "procedure" to follow to collect, process and interpret the information that will serve as the basis of knowledge. These "procedures" (technically called methods) are designed and used in order to give some "weight" or "strength" to the quality of the knowledge that is generated.

This does not mean that there are "hard-and-fast" rules which have to be memorized and applied all the time *stricto sensu*. This is a real big problem for research beginners. Understanding the application of different concepts in different situations requires much practice and some wits.

Experiences of some beginners in research

The following are just some of the worries of beginners in research at the very onset on their work: They ask themselves;

- What should the study be called? Is it a case-control? cohort? cross-sectional? longitudinal? prospective? or retrospective study?
- Which title is suitable?
- How best should the research hypothesis be formulated? (Perhaps the study might not require one!)
- What should the research questions be?
- What are the different parts of the "methods" section and how should it be written?
- Which statistical tests will be needed?
- Where do I get sufficient material for the literature review?
- How do I build a questionnaire or data collection sheet? Etc.

These questions preoccupy many students at the very onset of their research projects. Many spend time trying to arrange the title first, and then will want to clearly spell out the study objectives at the beginning of the study. This is a difficult thing to do especially if it is your very first try at research.

Believe it or not even the experienced at times have difficulties being as clear as print early on in research. They have an idea of what they want to do, get started and things become clearer as the work progresses. They then decide on what is most feasible and concentrate on this.

Two vital questions

Two fundamental questions will guide a beginner in research. Answers to these questions are keys to success in any research endeavor.

A. What do I want to do?
B. What is the best way to get it done?

You should first of all have a global idea of what you want to do. You may not be able to be very precise (no problem with that at this stage). However you should at least know the kind of people you may want to work with and what you will be measuring even if you cannot readily figure out how and with what (a little reading of other research works on similar topics will help).

Next, figure out how best this can be done (study design). Once you are clear about what you really want to do, go ahead and choose a design that is simple, straight-forward and feasible to answer the research questions. The title of the study and some other aspects can later be re-formulated at the end of the study. You do not decide first to carry out a randomized intervention and then try to formulate research questions and objectives that will suit this design. Often some cling onto a particular study design and then try to adjust every other thing to fit into this design. It may be a good and often ambitious design that is known to produce high quality evidence, but not the most appropriate to answer the research questions. So it is important knowing what you want to do first before deciding on how you may want to call it.

Getting started

Like any other profession or discipline, research has to be learned. You do not begin a career as a "*guru*". You learn the trade, gain experience and become mature. Expect complex situations that will require in-depth knowledge to solve. You will have to learn from each experience as the knowledge will be used in subsequent projects. Difficulties early on do not deter people who have a passion for something. Even some of the best of researchers have humble beginnings. Many can recall periods of sleepless nights over methodological puzzles, multiple rejections of manuscripts submitted for publication, satirical comments from journal peer-reviewers, and the list goes on. Somehow they pressed on and became masters of their art.

So how do you get started then? Just get a good idea, hang on to it and start working on it. For sure you will have many questions early on in your research project. You will especially have a hard time identifying and managing all potential sources of error in your study, especially with little or no experience in the art. But bear this in mind: *You will not always be able to answer all your questions at the beginning of the research project!*

This is because some things are sought out as the research project advances, based on what can be collected as information during the particular period of time with the available resources. Some circumstances beyond the control of the researcher can have sufficient impact on the focus of the research. So do not spend a lot of time trying to get all your questions answered before you begin. When you begin some questions will fall off your list while answers will show up for others. Especially, do not hesitate to ask for help from others with more knowledge and experience than yourself, or even from your peers. It is by rubbing your mind against other minds, especially those bigger than yours that you become sharper. Do not forget that research is more of team work. You will need the expertise of others.

If you encounter difficulties in research as a beginner rest assured that your concerns are genuine and that your fears are real, but more importantly there is a way out if only you can persevere and learn to look beyond those difficulties. You too can become a successful researcher or at least complete your dissertation or thesis in time after an enjoyable experience. There is always a starting point for any great adventure. It is my opinion that research is not the preserve of a selected few.

Can you figure the colorful front-page of a scientific journal with your name under the title of the article? Perhaps such a sight may stir you up.

Chapter Five

A novel self-help tool

Rationale for the research protocol

At the beginning of any research project you are expected to produce a document that explains all what you will do. This document is called a *research protocol*, and this is where it all begins. The research protocol is a guide or manual with a detailed plan of the research activities from start to finish. Often project supervisors may assist students by proposing research topics to them and then ask the student to write the research protocol.

But how do you produce a guide or manual on something you do not know much about? How and why should anyone expect you to write down the road-map to a place you don't know and have never been to? It is probably the very first time you have to carry out research. If you should write down what you are supposed to do before you actually do it implies that you already know how it is done or at least have an idea! That may sound crazy, and I know you agree with me. Probably *they* (supervisors) who have been into research before should rather write the research protocol while you suggest to them the topic you will like to work on.

Ok. No use lamenting over this. Maybe we can try to look at it this way. The life you live you have never lived it before. Yet you make plans for the future - a future that you can't see and don't know because you have never been there before. So you see, you simply *anticipate*. Does anticipating the future make any sense? It sure does, which is why you budget your finances, choose some careers over others, make some decisions at the expense of others, etc. So in writing a research protocol we can say that we are simply anticipating how we will achieve the set goals. Do you make changes in anticipated choices or decisions as life unfolds? The answer is yes. And so it is with research. It may happen that you have to make amendments to what was initially planned In the research protocol during execution of the project. Not everything is feasible.

Model template

But how do you *anticipate* in research and write down a protocol especially if you have never done so before? In this section we propose a way of doing it. We'll use a novel tool that is expected to guide the young researcher come up first with clear ideas on what s/he will do. Then further steps are presented to assist the amateur researcher think through the project. It is important to have an open mind and really be able to use your imagination. In that way you will generate your own ideas and write them down in your own words. This will prevent you from copying others.

The self-help tool encourages free and systematic thinking. The style is simple and straight-forward. This tool might be found particularly useful in settings where trainees do not receive sufficient assistance from academic staff, or for some healthcare providers interested in adding some research work to their daily routine of health care provision but who do not have the possibility of pursuing formal training. The points outlined in the template are sufficiently clear, with hints or clues for assistance. After using this template the student or beginner should be able to have a clearer picture of what he/she plans to do.

This novel tool is **not** intended to be a replacement for classical methods of learning research methods and does not attempt to summarize the complex domain of scientific research in seven steps. It is intended *to provide an opportunity for the beginner to "make sense" out of any research topic without much external help.*

The idea behind this tool is the assumption that as a beginner in research if you can successfully come up with a feasible and elaborate strategy that can permit you to correctly collect all the information required for your study, then you would have done the essential. You can always request for assistance when it comes to analyzing the collected information from those who master the art. Bear in mind also that data can be re-analyzed if the need arises. But no matter what complex and sophisticated data analysis procedures you employ, these cannot make up for poorly collected data. If you feed the computer software with data for analysis, it will run the analysis and produce results but these results can only be as good as the data you put in. If this data is "garbage" then the results can only be "garbage" despite the analysis techniques employed.

Finally the approach to research presented in this book is not specific or unique to research in the medical sciences but has been tailored to meet the needs of those in the medical and biomedical field making their debut in research.

Get ready for a thoughtful ride. Use your brain. Use your imagination. Just THINK!

Model Template

STEP 1
- What do you want to do exactly?
- Hint: Explain in very simple words such that somebody without a medical background should be able to understand you

STEP 2
- Where and when?
- Hint: Place and time period

STEP 3
- What group(s) of persons or documents do you intend to work with?
- Hint: Specifically define the characteristics of the individuals/groups of persons, or document types. ex. *All children aged between 2 months and 5 years in the pediatric ward with fever on admission*

STEP 4
- What do you plan to collect as information from them?
- Hint: Think logically from socio-demographic, clinical, laboratory, imaging, their opinion, etc

STEP 5
- What instrument(s)/tools will you use to collect these information?
- Hint: Think of the tools you will require to collect the information listed above, ex. *A mercury-in-glass thermometer for body temperature, a questionnaire to sample opinion*

STEP 6
- How will you use these instruments to collect the information you need?
- Hint: ex. *Place the bulb of the mercury-in-glass thermometer in the armpit of every participant for 5 minutes then record the reading on the data form*

STEP 7
- How will you get the potential participants to participate in your study OR how will you go about to select the necessary documents?
- Hint: You may have to invite them or go to where you can meet them, explain your aims and get consent, then recruit or assign as appropriate

Source: Tambe *et al*. BMC Medical Education (2014) 14:269

The model template ***does not*** oversimplify a complicated process but rather aims to put on course anyone making their first strides into research. It definitely does not perfectly fit some designs such as interventions and reviews. In this work technical words are used with care and attempts are made to explain what they mean in plain language.

Let us see how it works.

Seven Steps

STEP I. What do you want to do exactly?

Study aims or purpose

Answering this question requires that you *clearly* and simply state what you intend to do during the research. The statement should be straightforward and clear enough for just anyone to understand. The answer to this question will be the study *aims* or *purpose*.

A secret in being clear is to be able to say something using simple words such that any knowledgeable person without a medical background should be able to understand you.

Being clear and simple is not all that easy. It requires much thought, much effort, and much practice. The challenge you will have is to render scientific terminology and concepts into plain language for others to understand.

A simple and clear explanation does not mean that the concept or study to be undertaken is simple.

As the researcher you may understand yourself (or think you do!) but others do not understand you. After rendering the study aim in plain language you may then realize you probably never really understood what you would be doing during the research.

Being simple and clear in research is a result of ingenuity and hard work. You have to carefully and skillfully distill concepts to bring out readily understandable threads of information - and in plain language.

Model Example

After a two-month internship in the Pediatric department of a community hospital (let us call it CA Hospital), you observed that many of your patients in the pediatric emergency unit had fever and were subsequently admitted. Much of what you recall about your internship is the managing of fevers in children and so you are interested in finding out what this really represents as far as pediatric pathologies in that community hospital are concerned.

Somehow you start thinking that if it is something for which a solution is possible then you will have to show your findings to the health authorities so that they can take action. So you decided to carry out a study to find out the cause of these fevers and the impact on both the community and the patients. How can you put in plain language what you want to do (study aims)?

Let's try this out: "*to find out the proportion of children hospitalized in the pediatric emergency unit of CA hospital who had fever on admission during a given period and the possible causes of these fevers*". Do you realize how simple what you want to do can be stated? Care has been taken to avoid technical words as much as possible.

This way of stating the aim or purpose of a study does not require further explanation and gives any reader a global view of what the study is all about in plain language. Though this statement might be sufficient in presenting the aim or purpose of your study, it can be improved. The improvement will result in "objectives" which we will subsequently develop.

Research question(s)

This is(are) the question(s) your research project seeks to answer. In fact it is re-stating the aims or purpose of your study in the form of a question! From what we developed above the research questions of your study can be:

- *What is the proportion of hospitalized children in the pediatric emergency unit of CA Hospital who have fever on admission?*
- *What are the causes of the fevers?*

A good way to formulate a research question is to use the main aim of your research. This main aim is called the primary outcome. Please try to have just one primary outcome. It helps you avoid getting confused and mixed up. It is the one thing you should be able to say you achieved at the end of the study. This main outcome by itself may not give a complete picture and so other outcomes will have to be investigated. In the example we are using just knowing the proportion of fevers will definitely not be enough and so we also investigate on the causes of these fevers. Other secondary outcomes can be investigated such as living conditions, nutritional and vaccination status, schooling, use of insecticide-treated bed nets, laboratory findings, imaging findings, outcome after treatment, length of stay in the hospital, etc. Adding some secondary outcomes can help provide an explanation to what we observe primarily.

Research hypotheses

Does your study require a hypothesis? You should answer this question before delving for one. *But what is a hypothesis and how do I determine if my study requires one*?

Generally, a hypothesis is a "statement" that is made based on observations, experience or on facts generated by other studies concerning a particular concept. Why make this "statement"? This statement is what you will be studying in your research, to determine if it is true. So you will have to clearly state the "fact" you will be investigating and how you will determine if it is true or not.

Example:

Using the Model Example, say you probably had a lot of cases of fever in hospitalized children during your Pediatrics internship so much so that you came to conclude that close to 50% of the children admitted in that hospital during your internship had fever. But 50% is your subjective assessment. So you may want to check it further by consulting hospital records during a similar period to back up your assertion. Since you are already convinced that the proportion of admitted children in CA Hospital with fever is alarmingly high, you decide to formulate a "statement" that portrays this conviction and which you will seek to prove during your research. This "statement" (hypothesis) can be formulated thus:

The proportion of children admitted in the pediatric emergency unit of CA Hospital with fever on admission is at least 50%.

This statement (hypothesis) is supported by local hospital register data and not just your opinion, and so at least you have a basis for your conviction! This hypothesis is necessary because you have sufficient reason to be already convinced of the situation. If this were not the case such a statement would not be necessary and in the research you will be exploring to find out what the situation looks like and no hypothesis would be required!

You may want to compare the outcome of an event between two groups or two estimates in your research. Since you might not have any reason to believe that both outcomes should really be different, you can state that "*there is no difference between the groups or between the estimates*". Stating a hypothesis like this is called a *null hypothesis* (see Chapter Seven) because you are assuming there is no difference or no effect or no association (*null* means nothing, zero). The task of the study now will be to investigate if there is any difference between the estimates in question.

When a hypothesis is necessary, the basis for it should be explained with reference to the source of the fact. The hypothesis should be clearly stated and quantified, so that it will be possible to determine whether it is true.

Not all studies require a hypothesis.

If you rather would just want to explore a concept and find out what you can about it, then no need for a hypothesis! The results of your exploration would rather generate facts (hypotheses) that can be further tested in another study. So the decision to formulate a hypothesis depends on the aim of your study. If you want to confirm an assertion you will need one. If you want to explore to gather information, don't bother about one.

Do not force a hypothesis into your research project if none is necessary.

STEP II. Where and when?

Study setting and period

Where refers to the specific place(s) in which the study will be carried out, or at least for data collection. This is the "*study setting*". It could be a geographic location, neighborhood, school campus, place of work, etc. Most medical research are either hospital-based or community-based. Multiple settings may be involved.

When refers to the time frame for data collection and should be as precise as possible, say from the 1st of January to the 31st of December of a particular year (depending on what you plan to collect as information). This time frame is the "*study period*".

Model Example

- S*tudy setting*: this could be the *Pediatric emergency unit of CA hospital*
- *Study period*: from the 1st *of January to the 31st of December (year)*

We can now use this additional information to develop "*objectives*" for the *Model Example* as follows:

> "To find out the proportion of children hospitalized in the pediatric emergency unit of CA hospital from the 1st of January to the 31st of December (year) who had fever on admission"

Did you notice what was added? The study setting and period. Does this statement make more sense? It sure does!

We continue.

STEP III. What group(s) of persons and/or documents do you plan to work with?

Study participants

Not everybody in the general population may be of interest to your study and so you may want to work with a particular group of persons. What are the characteristics that define this group(s) of persons? These characteristics could be based on:

- Socio-demographic data: age, sex, nationality, occupation, marital status, place of residence or origin, ethnicity, education, income, etc.
- Clinical condition: particular clinical symptom(s), clinical state, event or disease.
- Para clinical profile; functional test(s) results, imaging or laboratory-based finding, etc.

More than one characteristic can define the group(s) of interest.

The group of persons you plan to work with is called the "*target population*". It is the pool of eligible participants from which you will recruit or select those who actually get to participate in the study.

Do not be in haste. Take time and think of all the most important features that should define the target population because all of the participants should share these features. The shared features that define this target population are called "inclusion/eligibility criteria".

You may not want to work with persons (this is not always possible) and so you may prefer to consult records/databases. The databases will have to be specified because different databases contain different kinds of information. You should be sure that the selected databases contain the kind of information you need.

Model Example

The target population could be:

"*All children aged from 2 to 59 months hospitalized in the Pediatric emergency unit of CA hospital during the specified study period*"

The definition of the target population in this example is based on *age* and *place of hospitalization*. However it may happen that some eligible persons identified for a study do not participate and so do not contribute to the data. The reasons that further rule out formerly eligible persons are termed "*exclusion criteria*".

In the *Model Example* all children less than 2 months or above 59 months of age, and those between 2 to 59 months of age hospitalized *elsewhere* in the hospital are not eligible. These are not exclusion criteria since these children do not fulfill the "conditions" to belong to the target population. However exclusion criteria will involve those children who are eligible but who for some reason cannot contribute to the data. (The reasons may include: informed consent not given by parent or guardian, incomplete data, drop-out from the study, etc).

Exclusion criteria are not non-inclusion criteria.

Study objectives

Putting together what we have gathered so far, we can formulate "*objectives*":

1. *To find out the proportion of children aged between 2 to 59 months hospitalized in the pediatric emergency unit of CA hospital who had fever on admission from the 1st of January to the 31st of December (year)*
2. *To determine the causes of the fevers in these children*
3. *To assess potential risk factors associated with febrile conditions in the study population*

These now read like real objectives.

Tips for formulating objectives

The acronym *S-M-A-R-T* is a helpful tool.

- *S: Specific.* Objectives should be sufficiently clear and target one thing at a time
- *M: Measurable.* Objectives should be measurable so that you can tell when they are met. They can be measured numerically, or could be a presentation of facts, opinion, etc
- *A: Achievable.* Objectives should be things that are practically possible to obtain with the selected study design
- *R: Relevant.* There should be a genuine reason for wanting to know this

- *T: Time-bound.* Objectives should be achievable within a given time frame

Research objectives should be what can actually be done with a genuine reason for wanting to do them and within a particular time frame using an appropriate study design.

Do not be too ambitious with your research objectives. Be realistic. Bear in mind also that occasionally objectives can be better formulated after data collection and analysis!

STEP IV. What do you plan to collect as information/data?

Variables

If you know what you specifically want to do it becomes easier to decide on what you will need as information to get it done. *The data to be collected will depend on what you set out to achieve as goal or objectives.*

This is not always easy. You will have to think logically. Take for example your primary objective and ask yourself, "If I have to attain this objective what do I need to collect as information?" Write these down. Do same for all the other objectives. Then also think of some other information that you will have to collect to enable you describe the study population.

Often in medical research the information collected usually includes but not limited to the following:

- Socio-demographic characteristics; age, gender, ethnicity, nationality, marital status, place of residence, occupation, level of education, income, etc.

These characteristics can be used to describe your sample and so anybody reading your work has an idea of the kind of persons you enrolled in your study. Try not to collect information that will really be of no use. If you have no reason to record participants' religion or ethnicity then don't.

- Clinical information: information on past health-related events, symptoms of disease, specific clinical conditions, findings on physical examination, clinical parameters such as body temperature, blood pressure, etc
- Laboratory measurements and imaging findings
- Views of participants, reported attitudes and practices, behaviors, etc.

These are some of the domains in which you will be collecting information often in your research. The list is not exhaustive and should only serve as a guide to help you think logically and design your data sheet to collect information following an ordered sequence. It will help you not to miss out on any vital information. Remember you will have to collect just what you will need to achieve your objectives.

This task is crucial and is not always easy as a beginner. You may have a hard time trying to figure out all what you might need as information. You have to be careful not to miss out on anything. You also have to be professional not to collect unnecessary information. However I think it is better to be a bit more exhaustive if you really do not know what will be relevant than to miss out on some important information, because you might not be able to get it again. As you gain more experience you will know with certainty from the beginning of your research what you will need as information so you won't have to collect irrelevant information that will have to be discarded.

Do some reading. What did other researchers measure? What can I add in my context? Will it be relevant?

Example

Let us consider the model example, what will be of interest to collect as information? Perhaps all of the following might be useful: Age, gender, schooling status, place of residence, vaccination status, type of feeding, blood group, Hemoglobin electrophoresis, use of insecticide-treated bed nets, previous admissions and diagnoses, surgeries, medications, known allergies and other medical ailments, symptoms on presentation and date of onset of each, findings on physical examination, body temperature, laboratory test results (full blood count, C–Reactive Protein, Erythrocyte sedimentation rate, blood smear test for malaria, etc), imaging findings (ultrasonography, chest radiograph, etc).

If you think constructively you will have a long list of variables for in-depth exploration of the situation. It is advisable to consult the literature and read on what has been done so far. Other works might inspire you as to what to include in your list of variables.

You now have a list of variables. Get sheets of paper and write down the variables, leaving spaces in which to fill in the value corresponding to each variable for each participant. You will then have to transfer these to a computer (Excel® spreadsheets or statistical software). It is always advisable to keep the hard copies of your data for some time.

STEP V. What instrument(s)/tools will you use to collect the information you need?

Study tools/equipment

Having a list of variables is important. Then ask "What will I need to collect each of this information?" Simply figure out how this can be done. For measurements you will have to specify the instruments to be used (instrument type, manufacturer, specifications, year of manufacture, etc). For example you might need a mercury-in-glass thermometer for body temperature, a weighing scale for weight, a mercury sphygmomanometer for blood pressure, a multi-detector computed tomography scanner if you want to assess findings in head trauma patients, etc. For surveys the key instrument is a questionnaire.

STEP VI. How will you use these instrument(s) to collect the information you need?

Study procedure

Measuring and recording of information during research is a delicate task as it can introduce errors in the data. Procedures will have to be standardized and performed in the same way for every participant in the study.

For measurements, ideally the same instrument or instrument type should be used where possible for every participant. The procedures will have to be written down and carefully followed for each participant. This is not easy when many investigators or volunteers are involved in measuring variables for study participants as differences are likely to be observed. Say for example five nurses are each measuring the brachial artery blood pressure of participants in a campaign to screen for arterial hypertension using oscillometric sphygmomanometers. You can be sure of variations in values even when the same nurse decides to take a second measurement for the same participant. These measurement *variations* can introduce sufficient errors which will affect overall results.

However, information for some variables will be available in electronic databases, some in medical records, for others you will have to interview participants or anybody who can give the required information. It will be necessary to test the tools to be sure they are accurate and can give correct results before starting to use them.

The recording of information is also delicate. It has to be precise and the same standard respected for all participants. The same units should be used for measurements, same precision (such as number of decimals), and same scale. The same questionnaire should be used for surveys. It will be important to pre-test questionnaires to clear any ambiguity.

Example

Say you want to measure the body temperature of children in a Pediatric ward. You will have to place the same kind of thermometer (say mercury-in-glass for example) in the same anatomic region for the same duration for every child!

If you do not know how an instrument is used, ask for help.

STEP VII. How will you get those who are eligible to participate in your study?

In order for the researcher to get individuals participate in their study they will have to identify potential study participants, devise a means of deciding who should participate if not all of them and get to meet potential candidates to invite them to do so.

This point embodies two principles in research: sampling and ethics. The following steps might be helpful:

- Advertise the study
- Go to where you can meet eligible participants

This might include hospital wards, specialized treatment centers, laboratories, schools, neighborhoods, etc. If that is not the convenient place for work you can later invite them to meet you at an appropriate environment, safe for both the participant and the researcher.

- Explain the study

When you approach potential participants, you'll have to clearly explain to them in plain language the aims of the study and the procedure. Potential threats of harm and any discomfort as a result of the procedure will have to be explained, with the measures taken to prevent them from happening. It is important for potential study participants to know that the study has been approved by the competent authorities (show proof of this by presenting the authorizations). The rights and responsibilities of participants during the study should be clear.

- Get consent

For those who will accept to participate in your study, let this acceptance be clearly expressed either verbally or through the signing of an informed consent form.

- Recruit or select.

Appropriately recruit participants who give consent to take part in the study. Study participants should be *representative* of the general population of interest and the number should be *reasonably large* to permit detection of differences.

Deciding on how to select participants for a study is known as *sampling*. Sampling is very important in research (like the study design) because errors introduced at this stage will definitely limit the use of the study findings. Given its importance, it is presented in more detail to permit a better understanding.

Sampling Methods

Volunteering: A study is advertised and people opt to participate.

Disadvantages: Generally people who opt are likely to be different in some way from people who do not. Perhaps they may be more knowledgeable about health issues and have different health-related behaviors, or very ill and so desperate for anything that might work.

Convenience sampling: Potential study participants are those who are easiest to reach or readily available to work with.

Disadvantages: Participants "conveniently" selected may not represent well the study target population, as their characteristics may be quite different from others. Say for example you want to find out the smoking habits of students in a university and you enroll only students from the faculty of health sciences because it is easier for you to reach them (and many of them are your friends since you are also a student of that faculty). The findings of your study may not apply to the entire university student community because students from the faculty of health sciences may likely have completely different smoking habits from students in other faculties that your study did not include and so your results remain valid only for the kind of participants you chose!

Consecutive sampling: Study participants are recruited as they come, on a first-come first-serve basis till a satisfactory number is reached.

Disadvantages: Only persons who present during the period of data collection will be studied. Study results can be affected by seasonal variations in disease occurrence or chance occurrences and can lead to false rates of disease.

Volunteering, convenience and consecutive sampling are likely to include study participants who are systematically different from other eligible persons who do not participate and will hence influence the study findings and result in "**bias**".

Random sampling

Simple random sampling: Participants are selected in a way that everyone has an equal chance of being selected. This is to avoid any conscious influence by the investigators over the choice of who gets to participate in a study. The selection of one participant does not influence the selection of another. To select a simple random sample, first of all get the sample frame; this is a list of all the eligible participants (could be a class list, telephone directory, list of house numbers in a street, hospital register, etc). Then assign an identification number to every entry, say from 1 to *N*. A table of random digits, computer software (Microsoft Excel®, Graphpad®, Research Randomizer®, etc) can be used to *randomly* select the required number of participants.

Disadvantages: It is not always possible to obtain a sample frame at the beginning of a study. Often when you carry out research you continuously recruit study participants as the study goes on so it is not always possible to have a list of all potential study participants at the beginning of your study! Also a simple random sample can completely miss out on some subgroups of the target population (termed *undercoverage*) resulting in a sample that is not representative of the general population of interest. To counteract this last problem, random samples can be stratified or systematized.

Stratified random sampling: The population of interest is divided into strata which could be defined by age, sex, ethnicity, etc depending on the type of study. A simple random sample is selected from each stratum and all the simple random samples are then put together. For example to select 10 students in a classroom known to have 100 students of which 40 are boys, a stratified random sample will be done such that amongst the 40 boys a simple random sample of 4 boys is selected and another simple random sample of 6 girls selected (from the 60 girls in the classroom), to finally produce a sample of 10 students that respects the sex ratio of the classroom. If stratification is not done a simple random sampling of the 100 students could lead to a selection of 10 students of which all could be boys or girls!

Systematic random sampling: A number assigned to an entry in the sample frame is first randomly selected, and then the other entries will be selected based on a defined rule, such as after every 10 or 20 entries thereafter.

Stratified and systematic random samples are not independent samples, because the selection of some participants is dependent on others.

Randomization

This term is most often used in intervention studies in which participants are assigned or allocated to different groups or arms in a study to receive an intervention *irrespective of how they were initially selected to participate in the study*. Participants can be volunteers or a convenience sample, but they are assigned or allocated *randomly* to any of the different groups in the study to receive the "pre-defined" intervention for the group. This is termed random assignment or random allocation. It is different from random sampling, which is used to refer to how participants are initially selected to participate in a study. It is important to understand this. Random assignment is done with aim to equally distribute prognostic factors in the participants in the different study groups and also to make the different groups comparable. The aim of such studies is not to infer findings to a general or theoretical population of interest as with simple random samples, but rather to measure the effects of an intervention.

Randomization can be simply done by assigning participants into different study groups irrespective of the number in each group (*simple randomization*). At times it is necessary to have an equal number of participants in each group and when this is done it is called *block randomization*.

It might not be possible to always randomly assign individual participants, often because the nature of the intervention does not permit this. So they are assigned as a "group" or "cluster", known as *cluster-randomization*. A cluster can be a doctor with all his clients or patients, a hospital with all the patients who come there, a family with all the members, a school or classroom with all the students in it, a neighborhood with all its residents, etc. "Units" with several individuals are randomized and not the individuals. That is if a family is assigned to receive a particular intervention, all the members of that family will receive that intervention.

Sampling methods are chosen based on the study design, objectives, and feasibility. There is no guarantee any sample will be "perfect" whatever the technique used. However it is important to understand the strengths and limitations of the various methods and also to what extent they can influence the findings of your study. Sample size calculations are not presented as the principles are profound to not permit a shallow summary. An article by Eng (2003) provides very useful information.[19]

Conclusion

After reading through this you should probably have a clue to some of the questions you have regarding your study. Hope you followed the sequence! At this point you might consider taking a break for some few minutes, drink some water, coffee or soft drink and feel some fresh air.

Want to continue? Ok. Just get some sheets of paper and write down your research topic if you already have one. If you don't, just figure out one now. Use the model template and think through the steps. Make sure you write down your thoughts because you might not be able to retrieve some great ideas that may cross your mind.

….

….

….

….

….

Through already? You now have the necessary material to comprehensively write up your research protocol. Let us see how those ideas can be arranged in the next chapter.

Chapter Six

Organizing ideas

Much has been done to help standardize the reporting of different types of studies. An example is the EQUATOR (*Enhancing the **QUA**lity and Transparency **Of** health **R**esearch*) network initiative which has produced reporting guidelines for different types of health research and these have been adopted by many editorial and review boards. There are recommendations for randomized trials, systematic reviews, observational studies, case reports, qualitative research, diagnostic studies, study protocols, etc. It is strongly recommended to use these proposed formats to present a research proposal/protocol or the findings of a study. The different documents are available at the equator network website www.equator-network.org.

It is also important to adhere to the particular style and preferences of your institution for dissertations and theses. In the section below some key elements to help organize ideas for the research proposal/protocol are presented briefly.

Title of the project

Give your project a "working title". This does not need to be the definitive title of your dissertation or thesis, just perhaps a description of what you intend to do during the project. This title should be concise and appropriately convey the concepts you plan to explore and the expected impact of the research. Write the names of the project investigators below the title or next page and identify the principal investigator (usually abbreviated PI). Provide supplementary information on the titles and/or academic ranks of the investigators/supervisors. Give the address (postal codes, e-mail address) of the investigators or at least the principal investigator and list institutional affiliations for all investigators.

Abstract

Provide a brief and concise summary of the entire project. The following structure can be used: Introduction and rationale, Objectives, Expected outcomes. About 250 to 300 words would suffice.

Description of the project

Introduction and Rationale

Present what you will be working on in the project. Explain why it is important to carry out the study. For example, why will it be important to know the reasons for admission in the pediatric unit of a community hospital? You need to defend the reason for the study and reference sources of information. It should be clear when you are stating your own ideas and when you are quoting someone else's. Let the flow of ideas be logical, leading the reader gradually to somewhere.

Aim(s)

State them here. You may have more than one aim so identify and write down the primary goal and some secondary goals if need be.

Research question(s) and hypotheses

State the research questions and hypothesis (if one is necessary for your study). Note that it is easy to do this by reformulating the specific study objectives as questions. It may require some tact to do this depending on the research topic.

Objectives

Clearly state the study objectives (be S-M-A-R-T). You can go back to the research questions to formulate each one as an objective.

Participants and Methods

Participants: Who is the target?

Study design: Give the choice of the selected study design and explain why this design was chosen (see chapter seven for study designs). Is it appropriate and feasible to answer the research questions? Will it generate high quality evidence? Is there a more appropriate design that could be used but which cannot be employed for some reasons? If so explain why.

Study setting and expected duration

Inclusion and exclusion criteria

Sampling

Explain the sampling method. You may also perform sample size calculations (if necessary!) Not every study will require this. Ask for expert advice if you are not sure.

Procedures

Describe in as much detail as possible all procedures, interventions, observations, measurements, instruments and how they will be used, etc. Anticipate potential adverse incidents and state how they might be dealt with.

Outcomes

What will be measured to directly provide answers to your study questions and/or research hypothesis? State the primary and secondary outcomes.

Data management and analysis

Say how collected data will be handled, verified, coded, monitored, stored, and protected. Computer programs to be used to analyze the data should also be stated. Anticipate statistical methods that will be employed to investigate each study objective and the necessary considerations to be made if any during the analysis. This section of the protocol will definitely not be the preferred for a beginner without much knowledge about statistics. Simply ask for advice from competent experts right from this stage of the work.

Ethics

Approvals from Ethics Committees and/or administrative clearance will be needed. If you know of the institutions then state where the protocol will be submitted and the administrative authorizations that may be necessary. How will informed consent be obtained? Will it be necessary at all, verbal and/or written?

How confidentiality and anonymity of participants' information will be ensured during the study will have to be discussed. Other issues that will have to be addressed include the rights of participants during the study, management of potential threats of harm during and after the study.

Project management

Roles

The roles of the investigators should be clear. Who will do what? Collaboration with other researchers and institutions should be stated and their expected input.

Write out everything that might be needed, from pens, pencils, sheets of paper, notebooks, computers, printers, telephones, clinical, laboratory and imaging equipments, offices, conference halls, etc.

Budget

Make a comprehensive budget for the project. It should be reasonable if you intend to apply for funding.

Example:

Items	Estimated cost
Office equipment (papers, pens, pins, computers, charts, etc)	…$
Diagnostic equipment	…$
Work facilities, office space, etc	…$
Transportation	…$
Accommodation	…$
Incentives; participants, volunteers, staff, etc	…$
etc	…
Total	…$

Time frame

Present a timetable of proposed activities that you plan to carry out and the estimated time frame for each activity. The following is an example of a time frame:

Activities	Timeline (weeks)	Deadline
Develop protocol	4	31 Jan 20--
Submit to supervisor for comments	2	14 Feb 20--
Update protocol based on supervisor's comments	2	28 Feb 20--
Submit protocol for ethical clearance	8	
Advertise study (if necessary)	2	
Pilot phase	2	
Adjustments after pilot phase	1	
Data collection	16	
Data analysis	1	
Data interpretation	1	
Manuscript writing	1	
Obtain corrections from supervisor	4	
Update manuscript based on supervisor's comments	1	
Submit corrected version for further comments	2	
Final corrections	2	
Writing of article and submitting for publication	2	
Presentation of findings to stakeholders	2	

You may consider using a Gantt chart to present the time frame of activities instead of a table.

Anticipated problems

Any anticipated difficulty should also be noted.

Information products and use

The main information product could be a dissertation or thesis to be defended publicly, or just a project report. You may also consider writing articles or publishing a book to improve visibility and further disseminate the findings of your research. But who will use the findings of your study? It is usually important to identify potential stakeholders before the study begins and present to them the study protocol. By engaging them from the start they will likely value the findings and that will give the project more credibility.

Remember, the aim of a study is to generate information. But this information will have to be converted to knowledge and applied!

Referencing

Write down the list of all documents cited in the work. Verify the accuracy of all citations. Write down the references *consistently* whatever style you choose or as recommended by your institution or journal. Computer software for referencing can be used such as *Reference Manager®, EndNote®, Mendeley®, Zotero®*, etc.

Tips for referencing

- Be consistent, whatever style you choose.
- *Number of authors*; some prefer you cite the first 3 or first 6 authors if more than 6 followed by *et al*.
- *Authors' names and initials*. Write the family name and the initial of the first and middle names for all the authors.

- *Journal name*: Should all be written in full or abbreviated using the official abbreviation (you can verify this online at *Index Medicus*).
- *Punctuation*: Note the positions of commas, semi-colons and colons. Also take note of where there are spaces and no spaces! If anybody wants to do a quick check of your reference list be sure this is where they will easily get you.
- *Issue numbers* for journal articles (usually written in brackets after the volume number) should be written for all references or omitted in all. Follow the journal or institutional recommendations on whether to include them or not.
- *Page numbers*: Either write as *123-128* for all of the references or *123-8*.
- Do not forget to state the date electronic sources were accessed.

NB: Softwares have come to make this tedious process easy. Divers output styles are readily available and many journal-specific preferences have been incorporated in many softwares. It is important to still understand that being consistent is key.

Annexes

These are supporting documents for the project. At this stage of the work you would just have a sample data form or questionnaire and the informed consent form. At the end of the project you would have to include in your report other supporting documents such as ethical approvals, authorization(s), maps, organizational charts, picture charts, flow diagrams of processes, photographs of equipments, etc.

Chapter Seven

Appraising evidence

When reading through any piece of scientific work or when checking through your own work you should be able to critically appraise the quality of the work and assess the strength of the evidence. This will determine the degree of confidence you can place on the results and the extent to which you will be willing to apply the evidence in your practice. The EQUATOR network has great tools for appraisal (www.equator-network.org).

1. Research question(s), hypotheses; are they clear?

This is where it all begins. Are the research questions clearly stated? The research hypothesis(es) if required should be well formulated and quantified. See Chapter Five.

2: Study design; appropriate?

You should then determine if the selected study design is the most appropriate and feasible design to answer the research questions or to test the hypothesis. In medical research often health and disease conditions are studied in human populations – aspects studied include the "distribution" and "determinants" of these conditions. Distribution classically refers to person, place and time attributes ("who", "where" and "when"). Determinants refer to "why" the condition occurs and "how". Studying health and disease conditions is termed "epidemiology". Epidemiology and biostatistics are fundamental disciplines in medical research. A summary of study designs is presented subsequently.

Epidemiologic study designs

Generally, study designs can be classified either as:

1. *Descriptive* (address the questions "who", "where" and "when") and *Analytic* (address the questions "why" and "how"); or
2. *Observational* (descriptive + analytic) and *Experimental* (analytic)

For consistency with the concept of "distribution and determinants" of health and disease conditions, we will adopt the distinction between descriptive and analytic study designs. The table below illustrates.

Table 7.1 - Study designs

Descriptive study designs	Analytic study designs
	Observational
• Case report	• Cohort
• Case series	• Case-control
• Cross-sectional (surveys)	Experimental
• Correlational	• Randomized Interventions
	• Non randomized Interventions

Case report: Comprehensive description of the experience of a single individual.

Case series: Focused description of individuals with some similar condition.

Cross-sectional studies (or surveys): Assess an outcome of interest at a given point in time. No causal link can be made since the outcome of interest and potential causes are measured at the same time.

Correlational studies: Concerned with the relationship between variables in entire populations as a whole and not in individuals.

Cohort studies: Persons with a similar characteristic (cohort) are followed up and specific outcomes are recorded after a period of time. Participants are initially classified based on whether they receive a particular exposure or not, and the occurrence of the outcome of interest is compared between the exposed and the unexposed groups. Ever heard of *Relative Risk*?

Case-control studies: Participants are enrolled based on the presence of a particular health-related event or disease (cases). Some other persons without the health-related event or disease (controls) and who are similar in other characteristics to those with the condition (such as age, sex, ethnicity, socioeconomic status, etc) are also enrolled. Both groups are interviewed about past specific exposures and the occurrence of these exposures between the cases and the controls are compared. Do you know about *Odds Ratios*?

Intervention studies: Participants are assigned to receive a pre-determined intervention (randomly or not) or to serve as a control (no intervention received). Some pre-defined outcome measures are then compared between those who received the intervention and those who did not. Clinical trials are just one type of intervention studies. Whatever study design is used the choice has to be explained.

Retrospective and prospective: These terms do not refer to a particular study design *per se* but are rather descriptive attributes. Generally they are used to describe data collection with respect to the occurrence of an outcome. A study is described as retrospective if at the time data is collected both the exposure and the outcome of interest have already occurred, and prospective if the outcome has not yet occurred. For example, in case-control studies participants are interviewed to find out specific exposures that may be associated with an outcome of interest. Given that disease (the outcome) has already occurred before the study begins, case-control studies are retrospective studies.

Longitudinal: This is another descriptive attribute which refers to studies in which subjects are followed-up over time with continuous and/or repeated measurements.

3: Methods; well described?

After checking on the selection of an appropriate study design, the methods have to be carefully checked. The target population has to be well defined. Inclusion and exclusion criteria, sampling method and sample size, study period and duration, instruments, procedures and study outcomes have to be clearly explained. Check for appropriateness and feasibility of all these. Safety precautions, ethical considerations, data collection, management and analysis have to be screened.

4: Data presentation; correct summary statistics?

Is the data appropriately summarized and presented? What measures of central tendency and spread are presented? Is the data normally distributed or skewed? Here are some of the principles on how to summarize and present data.

Data are summarized using the center (middle values) and the spread (dispersion). Measures which indicate the center of a distribution of data are the mean (average value), median (middle value) and the mode (most frequent value). The spread is assessed using the range, interquartile range, standard deviation, standard error, and the coefficient of variation.

Measures of central tendency

Mean

The arithmetic mean is the average value of a number of observations. It is used to describe the center of a normal distribution. Because it is an average it is sensitive to extreme values (outliers). The geometric mean is calculated after logarithmic transformation of the values of observations and used to describe this data set because the logarithms of the observations are normally distributed. The geometric mean is particular useful to summarize laboratory data.

Median

This is the value of the central observation after all the observations have been ordered from the least to the greatest or vice versa. It is unaffected by extreme values (outliers) and is a more informative summary statistic if the distribution is skewed (asymmetric).

Mode

This is the value that occurs most often in a set of data and can provide insights into possible causes of disease.

Measures of spread (dispersion)

Range

This is the difference between the maximum and the minimum values of a data set.

Percentiles

Divide the data into 100 equal parts. The pth percentile is the value that has p percent of the observations falling at or below it.

Quartiles

These divide a data set into four equal parts. Each part (quartile) has 25% of the data. The first quartile (Q1) has 25% of all the data below it, Q2 has 50% of the data below it also and Q3 has 75% of the data below it. (Q2 = P50 = median)

Interquartile range (IQR)

It represents the central portion of the distribution, that is, from the first to the third quartiles Q1 to Q3, or 25th to the 75th percentile. IQR measures the spread of data around the median.

Standard deviation (SD)

SD gives an idea of the variability of the different observations around the mean. It estimates how close or how far the observations are from the center.

Standard error

It refers to the variability in the distribution of an estimate if *repeated samples* are drawn from a given population. If you draw many samples from a population, you will likely have a different value for an estimate (say the mean) for each sample, and this gives rise to a sampling distribution. The equivalence of a 'standard deviation' of this *sampling* distribution is called the standard error. For the mean, the standard error (SE) is estimated by dividing its standard deviation by the square root of the number of observations (n); $SE = SD/\sqrt{n}$. SE is used to calculate confidence intervals and test statistics for statistical inference.

Coefficient of variation

The coefficient of variation is used to compare the variability of estimates of distributions that differ in their units of measurement. Coefficient of variation, CV = (SD/mean) × 100%.

Presenting data: mean ± SD or median (range or IQR)?

If the data is normally distributed the mean and SD should be used, often expressed as mean ± SD. If the data is asymmetrical or skewed, the median and range or inter-quartile range should be presented; median (IQR) or median (minimum – maximum).

5: What measures of disease frequency and association?

Measures of disease frequency

Prevalence (P) is the proportion of the number of existing cases of a disease at a given point in time. Prevalence expresses the probability of being ill at the point in time being studied. Two types can be distinguished, point and period prevalence.

Incidence (I) is the number of new cases of a disease occurring during a specified period of time in a population at risk. Incidence expresses the risk of becoming ill. There are two types: cumulative incidence and incidence rate or incidence density.

Case fatality: This is the proportion of deaths amongst persons diagnosed with a disease in a given period. It expresses disease severity.

Mortality rates: Express the proportion of deaths during a specified period in a given population. Specific rates can be used (e.g. age group, gender).

Measures of association

These are statistics that quantify the relationship between variables.

Relative risk (risk ratio): It is the ratio of the incidence of disease among the exposed to the incidence of disease among the unexposed.

Odds ratio (OR): It is the ratio of the odds of exposure among those with disease (cases) to the odds of exposure among those without disease (controls).

Measures of impact

These quantify the expected impact if a particular variable is suppressed.

Risk difference, excess risk or attributable risk: This is the difference in the incidence rates of disease between the exposed and unexposed.

Attributable fraction (%) = risk difference × 100/incidence among the exposed population.

6: Role of chance, bias, and confounding addressed?

In assessing evidence from research the effect of some factors have to be considered.

Chance

Findings in studies can be due to some unknown and unpredictable factors which cannot be controlled for. Reported statistical associations can be due to such factors and not necessarily the variables being studied.

Bias

This is anything that influences the results, causing the reported estimates to be systematically different from what could be expected. There are many different ways in which study results can be influenced. The best known of which are selection bias, that is the study participants are systematically different from those who did not participate in the study, and measurement bias, which has to do with all the possible errors introduced when measuring variables and assessing outcomes.

Confounding

This is the distortion of the relationship between an "exposure" and an "outcome" of interest due to an extraneous variable that is related to both the "exposure" and "outcome" variables. Such "relationship-distorting" variables are referred to as confounders and they influence the measured effect between the dependent and the independent variables in an experiment. It is not always easy to identify or control for confounders, but they can be controlled for in many ways. In the study design, the following can be done: random sampling or random assignment, restriction of studies to persons with particular characteristics and matching cases with controls for some characteristics. At the analysis stage stratification can be done (analysis amongst different groups or strata) and multivariate models can be used.

When appraising any study or yours try to think of all possible sources of error and check if they were appropriately addressed.

7: Statistical tests

It is always important to check on the statistical tests used to assess outcomes to check if they are the most appropriate. The tests will depend on the hypotheses to be tested, associations and relationships between variables to be assessed and the type of variables. It is advisable to consult with a statistician or a researcher versed with statistical methods for data analysis if inexperienced.

8: Data interpretation

Tests of hypotheses

In many articles there are tests of hypotheses with associated probability values. It is important to understand the principle of statistical inference to be able to make sense out of such results.

During research we do not work with the entire population of interest because this is not practically possible. So we carefully select a subset called a sample. It has to be sufficiently large and representative of the population of interest from which it is drawn. A sufficiently large sample will give the statistical tests sufficient 'power' to detect differences. If the sample is selected to be representative (though we really do not have any guarantee of that) then we would want to extend the findings of the study to this population of interest. (Some rather prefer a theoretical distribution to population)

Often in research the aim is not to limit the findings to the individuals studied but to extend the findings from these individuals studied to the bigger population from which they were drawn. The process of 'extending' the findings from a sample to a bigger 'population' from which the sample was drawn is called inference. In quantitative research statistical methods are used for this process and so it is called statistical inference.

For a reminder, sample estimates are called *statistics* while population estimates are called *parameters*. So the mean of a sample is a *statistic* ($\bar{x}$) while the mean of a population is a *parameter* (μ; which is often unknown and therefore estimated from the sample mean, $\bar{x}$).

Say we obtain an estimate in a sample (a statistic):

What is the chance that an individual in the larger population of interest who was not part of our sample will have a value for this estimate that is similar or not considered to be significantly different from what we obtained?

For example if the mean age of women in our sample is 30 years, what is the chance that if we go back to the population of interest and randomly select a woman who did not participate in our study her age will not be significantly different from the 30 years we obtained? To determine this we make use of some probability concepts. (*NB: "Significant" in statistics would mean probably true, or not due to chance.*)

Consider the normal probability density plot below. The total area under the curve represents the sum of probabilities, and this is equal to 1 or 100%.

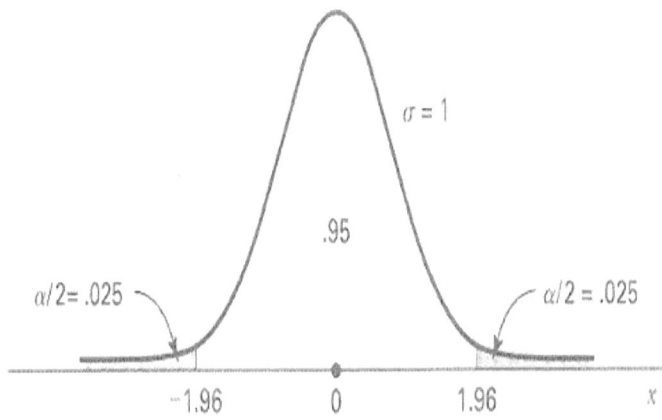

Source: https://onlinecourses.science.psu.edu/stat509/node/37

Practically we cannot be 100% sure that our sample statistic perfectly reflects the population parameter and so we select a cut-off. The cut-off or threshold in this figure is 5% or 0.05 and this is represented by the shaded areas as both sum up to 5% (0.025 + 0.025). All the calculated probabilities that fall within the non shaded area represented here as the portion between -1.96 to +1.96 are interpreted to mean that there is no considerable or significant difference or association between the estimates being compared. These probability values are greater than 5% or 0.05. Probabilities that lie within the shaded area are values less than 5% (< 0.05) and presented here as the 'rejection region'. These probabilities less than 0.05 are interpreted to mean there is a considerable or significant difference or association between the estimates being compared. This probability is also called a 'p value'.

So let us say we are comparing our sample statistic with a "theoretical value".

What is the chance that our sample statistic is not considered significantly different from this theoretical value?

Or

How well does our sample statistic predict this theoretical value?

If the probability of both estimates being similar is computed and found to lie in the non shaded area of the normal probability density plot ($p > 5\%$ or 0.05), we will interpret this probability by saying that there is no significant difference between the estimates. (The sample statistic will likely reflect the theoretical value). If the probability of both estimates being similar or associated is computed and found to lie in the shaded area of the normal probability density plot ($p < 5\%$ or 0.05), we will interpret this probability by saying that there is a significant difference between both estimates. (The sample statistic does not reflect theoretical value). Because we are using statistical methods to make inference the terminology would be improved by adding the adverb 'statistically' in interpreting the probability values. So a $p < 0.05$ would mean a statistically significant difference or association while a $p > 0.05$ would mean no statistically significant difference or association.

The null hypothesis

There is a concept that is implied in the above explanation of inference – the null hypothesis. We developed the above explanation based on the premise that there is "no difference" or "no association" between the estimates concerned. This initial premise of "no difference" or "no association" is a *null* hypothesis (*null* means zero, nothing). Otherwise stated the difference between the estimates is zero, or nothing (e.g $a - b = 0$, which is same as writing $a = b$). On the other hand there might be a "difference" between the two estimates and this situation will be called the *alternate* hypothesis. So either there is no difference or no association between estimates (null hypothesis) or there is a difference (alternate hypothesis). "No difference" or "no association" means that any observed difference is attributed to chance.

To summarize, if $p < 0.05$ (belonging to the shaded area of the normal probability density plot) then there is a statistically significant difference or association between the estimates and the null hypothesis of "no difference" or "no association" is rejected (remember this shaded area is the rejection area). So we conclude that there is an important difference or association between the estimates and we may later try to find out possible explanations for this difference. If the $p > 0.05$ (belonging to the non shaded area), we conclude that there is no statistically significant difference or association between the estimates and the null hypothesis of "no difference" or "no association" cannot be rejected. This second interpretation sounds complicated! The question you may ask is: "*If we do not reject the null hypothesis, why don't we accept it?*" This would be a logical position. It is important to understand the reporting. If you cannot reject the null hypothesis (as you would readily do when $p < 0.05$) do not say that it is accepted. It is actually difficult to truly demonstrate "no difference" or "no effect" from a small one. It is also statistically not possible to determine that there is "no difference". We are simply working on probabilities with the ever looming threat of being wrong.

Take note that a very small p value does not completely exclude the role of chance (it could be due to bias and confounding also). Probabilities express the likelihood of an event occurring and there is usually the possibility we might be wrong, however small. Also, statistically significant findings are not always clinically significant or relevant.

Confidence intervals (CI)

CIs are very important. They are calculated for sample estimates (statistics) but the ultimate goal is to give a range of values or "interval" in which we expect the true value to lie. To interpret a 95% CI result, we can say that there is a 95% chance that the true value for the estimate lies in that range. CIs can be calculated for proportions, relative risks, odds ratios, etc.

Investigating hypotheses using CIs

Firstly write down the null hypothesis, then have a look at the computed CI. If the value of the statistic for which the null hypothesis is true lies within the interval, then we say any observed difference or association is not statistically significant and so we cannot reject the null hypothesis.

Example

Say the *difference* d between two means or proportions is expressed as a CI, that is $d = 2.5$ (-1 to 5). The expression in brackets refers to the CI. The null hypothesis of "no difference" is that the *difference* d between these means or proportions is zero (i.e. $d = 0$). The value of d for which the null hypothesis is true is 0, and this value is comprised within the reported CI (0 is included in the interval -1 to 5). We therefore cannot reject the null hypothesis and therefore say that the difference between the means or proportions is not statistically significant. (*What if the CI was 1.5 to 5?*)

Conversely if the value of the statistic for which the null hypothesis is true is out of the interval, then we conclude that the observed difference or effect is statistically significant and the null hypothesis is rejected.

Example

Let us assume that in a study lung cancer was found to be associated with cigarette smoking, and the reported statistic is the odds ratio (OR) which is presented as 20 (17 - 22). A null hypothesis of "no association" will be that there is no association between lung cancer and cigarette smoking. For the null hypothesis to be true then OR should be = 1. We already have the estimated CI, 17 to 22. As a matter of fact, the value of the statistic is always within the CI! The value of the OR for the null hypothesis to be true is 1 and this value is out of the interval 17 to 22, so we conclude that there is a significant association (and not difference giving that we are dealing with an association here) between lung cancer and smoking. The null hypothesis is therefore rejected.

Coming back to the example on the difference between two means or proportions, if this was reported as 2.5 (1.5 to 5) then the value of the statistic for the null hypothesis to be true ($d = 0$) is out of the CI range and this difference is now interpreted as being statistically significant. The null hypothesis of "no difference" is rejected.

9: Study conclusion(s) based on findings or intuitive?

Are the conclusions of the study based on the data actually reported? This is necessary to verify because sometimes conclusions can be made intuitively. Is there any attempt to link the conclusion to the study aim or objectives? It is also possible that study conclusions are completely isolated from the aim of the study leaving the reader to wonder what the study was all about.

10: Your own conclusion

Conclude on the quality of the study: the research questions and hypothesis, the type of participants and methods, and the study findings. Did the study actually investigate what it purported? Is the quality acceptable? Can the findings be used in your setting? If no, what are the aspects limiting your use of it?

Beware of exaggerated reporting of associations and significance test results, or their anticipated impact. Study the data and draw the conclusion yourself. If you can do this then you can be sure of objectively assessing scientific evidence. Also if your own work can go through this process then you will be able to produce quality research.

Remember, quality does not mean a "perfect" paper. Usually studies have some limitation(s) and it is scientific to appropriately address these.

Bibliography

1. Wickramasinghe DP, Perera CS, Senarathna S, Samarasekera DN. Patterns and tends of medical student research. *BMC Med Educ.* 2013;13:175.
2. Detsky MED, Detsky AS. Encouraging medical students to do research and write papers. *CMAJ.* 2007;176:1719-1721.
3. Rivera JA, Levine RB, Wright SM. Completing a scholarly project during residency training: Perspectives of residents who have been successful. *J Gen Intern Med.* 2005;20:366–369.
4. Munung NS, Vidal L, Ouwe-Missi-Oukem-Boyer O. Do students eventually get to publish their research findings? The case of Human Immunodeficiency Virus/Acquired Immunodeficiency Syndrome research in Cameroon. *Ann Med Health Sci Res.* 2014;4:436–441.
5. Nieminen P, Sipilä K, Takkinen HM, Renko M, Risteli L. Medical thesis as part of the scientific training in basic medical and dental education: experiences from Finland. *BMC Med Educ.* 2007;7:51.
6. Salmi LR, Gana S, Mouillet E. Publication pattern of medical theses, France, 1993-98. *Med Educ* 2001;35:18-21.
7. Sipahi OR, Caglayan SD, Pullukcu H, et al. Publication rates of Turkish medical specialty and doctorate theses on Medical Microbiology, Clinical Microbiology and Infectious Diseases disciplines in international journals. *Mikrobiyol Bul.* 2014;48:341-345.
8. Saldaña-Gastulo JJ, Quezada-Osoria CC, Peña-Oscuvilca A, Mayta-Tristán P. High frequency of plagiarism in medical theses from a Peruvian public university. *Rev Peru Med Exp Salud Publica.* 2010;27:63-67.
9. Salgueira A CP, Gonçalves M, Magalhães E, Costa MJ. Individual characteristics and student's engagement in scientific research: a cross-sectional study. *BMC Med Educ.* 2012;12:95.

10. Frishman WH. Student research projects: should they be a requirement for medical school graduation? *Heart Dis.* 2001;3:140-144.
11. Sheikh FQS, Sheikh AS, Kaleem A, Waqas A. Factors contributing to lack of interest in research among medical students. *Adv Med Educ Pract.* 2013;4:237-243.
12. Tambe J, Ze Minkande J, Moifo B, Ongolo-Zogo P, Mbu R, Gonsu J. Students' perspectives on research and assessment of a model template designed to guide beginners in research in a medical school in Cameroon. *BMC Med Educ.* 2014;14:269.
13. Burgoyne LN, O'Flynn S, Boylan GB. Undergraduate medical research: the student perspective. *Med Educ Online.* 2010;15:10.
14. Siemens DR, Punnen S, Wong J, Kanji N. A survey on the attitude towards research in medical school. *BMC Med Educ.* 2010;10:4.
15. Hren D, Lukic K, Marusic A, et al. Teaching research methodology in medical schools: students' attitudes towards and knowledge about science. *Med Educ.* 2004;38:81-86.
16. Vujaklija A, Hren D, Sambunjak D, et al. Can teaching research methodology influence students' attitude toward science? Cohort study and nonrandomized trial in a single medical school. *J Investig Med.* 2010;58:282-286.
17. Saunders J. The practice of clinical medicine as an art and as a science. *Med Humanities.* 2000;26:18–22.
18. Panda SC. Medicine: Science or Art? *Mens Sana Monogr.* 2006;4:127–138.
19. Eng J. Sample size estimation: How many individuals should be studied? *Radiology.* 2003;227:309-313.

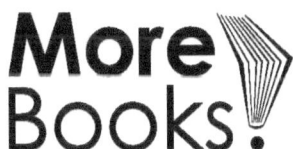

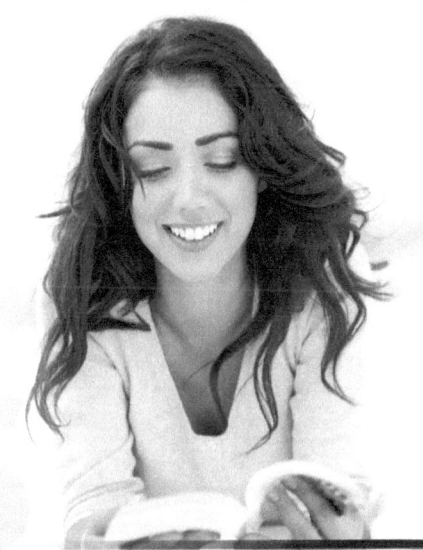

I want morebooks!

Buy your books fast and straightforward online - at one of the world's fastest growing online book stores! Environmentally sound due to Print-on-Demand technologies.

Buy your books online at

www.get-morebooks.com

Kaufen Sie Ihre Bücher schnell und unkompliziert online – auf einer der am schnellsten wachsenden Buchhandelsplattformen weltweit! Dank Print-On-Demand umwelt- und ressourcenschonend produziert.

Bücher schneller online kaufen

www.morebooks.de

OmniScriptum Marketing DEU GmbH
Heinrich-Böcking-Str. 6-8
D - 66121 Saarbrücken
Telefax: +49 681 93 81 567-9

info@omniscriptum.com
www.omniscriptum.com

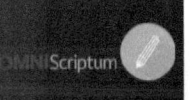

www.ingramcontent.com/pod-product-compliance
Chambersburg PA
CBHW020455220526
45464CB00002B/998